Preventing
Child Sexual Abuse Within
Youth-serving Organizations:

Getting Started on Policies and Procedures

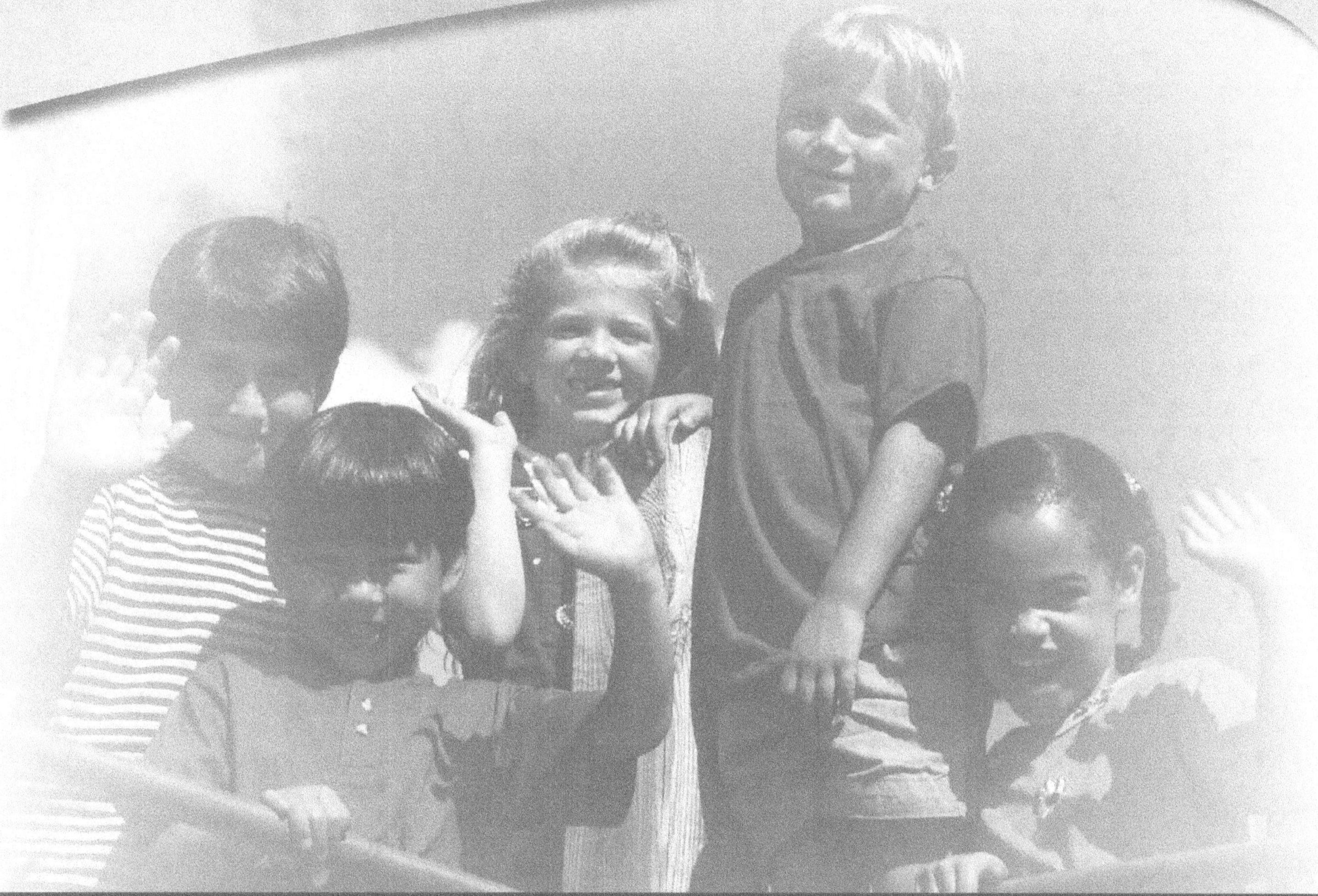

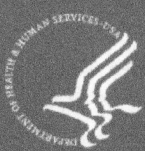

U.S. DEPARTMENT OF HEALTH AND HUMAN SERVICES
Centers for Disease Control and Prevention

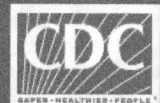

Preventing Child Sexual Abuse Within Youth-serving Organizations: Getting Started on Policies and Procedures

U.S. DEPARTMENT OF HEALTH AND HUMAN SERVICES
Centers for Disease Control and Prevention
National Center for Injury Prevention and Control
Division of Violence Prevention
Atlanta, Georgia

2007

Preventing Child Sexual Abuse Within Youth-serving Organizations: Getting Started on Policies and Procedures is a publication of the National Center for Injury Prevention and Control of the Centers for Disease Control and Prevention.

Centers for Disease Control and Prevention
Julie L. Gerberding, M.D., M.P.H., Director

Coordinating Center for Environmental Health and Injury Prevention
Henry Falk, M.D., M.P.H., Director

National Center for Injury Prevention and Control
Ileana Arias, Ph.D., Director

Division of Violence Prevention
W. Rodney Hammond, Ph.D., Director

Suggested citation: Saul J, Audage NC. *Preventing Child Sexual Abuse Within Youth-serving Organizations: Getting Started on Policies and Procedures.* Atlanta (GA): Centers for Disease Control and Prevention, National Center for Injury Prevention and Control; 2007.

Authors

Janet Saul, Ph.D.
Division of Violence Prevention
National Center for Injury Prevention and Control

Natalie C. Audage, M.P.H.
Consultant and former ASPH/CDC Fellow

Acknowledgements

The authors would like to acknowledge the individuals and organizations that participated in the meeting of experts sponsored by CDC in August 2004. The authors would also like to thank Kristin Leydig Bryant for facilitating the meeting and Deborah A. Ausburn, Attorney at Law, for reviewing the document.

Table of Contents

Introduction 1

Components of Child Sexual Abuse Prevention 3
    Screening and selecting employees and volunteers 4
    Guidelines on interactions between individuals...9
    Monitoring behavior...13
    Ensuring safe environments...15
    Responding to inappropriate behavior, breaches in policy, and allegations
        and suspicions of child sexual abuse 17
    Training about child sexual abuse prevention 22
        Training employees/volunteers...24
        Training caregivers 27
        Training youth..28

Overcoming Challenges to Child Sexual Abuse Prevention in
        Youth-serving Organizations 29

Conclusion: Moving Forward 33
    Organizational processes for developing and implementing child sexual abuse
        prevention policies...33
    Child sexual abuse prevention planning tool for organizations..........................35

Appendixes

Appendix A: Participant List 39

Appendix B: Resource List and Sample Policies 42
    Books/Publications/Videos/Workshops 42
    Journal articles 47
    Sample policies from participating organizations 47
    Publications with sample policies and procedures 48
    Relevant organizations...49

Introduction

Youth-serving organizations strive to create a safe environment for youth, employees, and volunteers so that youth can grow, learn, and have fun. Part of creating a safe environment is making sure that youth are not harmed in any way while participating in organization-sponsored activities. One risk in any organization working directly with youth is child sexual abuse.

It is vital that organizations create a culture where child sexual abuse is discussed, addressed, and prevented.

This report is designed for representatives of youth-serving organizations who are interested in adopting strategies to prevent child sexual abuse. Whether these strategies are developed within the context of an overall risk management plan or are addressed separately, organizations need to examine how they can protect youth from sexual abuse.

Definitions

- Children and youth
  - Anyone between the ages of zero and 17 years. In this document, these terms are used interchangeably.

- Child sexual abuse
  - "Child sexual abuse involves any sexual activity with a child where consent is not or cannot be given. This includes sexual contact that is accomplished by force or threat of force, regardless of the age of the participants, and all sexual contact between an adult and a child, regardless of whether there is deception or the child understands the sexual nature of the activity. Sexual contact between an older and a younger child also can be abusive if there is a significant disparity in age, development, or size, rendering the younger child incapable of giving informed consent. The sexually abusive acts may include sexual penetration, sexual touching, or non-contact sexual acts such as exposure or voyeurism."[1]
  - Legal definitions vary by state, so look up your state guidelines using the Child Welfare Information Gateway (www.childwelfare.gov/systemwide/laws_policies/search/index.cfm).

What You Will Find in This Report

In the first section, you will find six key components of child sexual abuse prevention for organizations. These components were identified by the Centers for Disease Control and Prevention (CDC) in conjunction with experts:

1. Screening and selecting employees and volunteers
2. Guidelines on interactions between individuals
3. Monitoring behavior
4. Ensuring safe environments
5. Responding to inappropriate behavior, breaches in policy, and allegations and suspicions of child sexual abuse
6. Training about child sexual abuse prevention.

---

[1]Myers JEB, Berliner L, Briere J, Hendrix CT, Jenny C, Reid TA, editors. *The APSAC handbook of child maltreatment.* 2nd ed. Thousand Oaks (CA): Sage Publications; 2002. p. 55.

Each component is described in detail, including the prevention goals, critical strategies, and additional strategies that could be considered depending on the context and resources of individual organizations.

The sections that follow offer suggestions for addressing challenges to developing and implementing a strategy to prevent child sexual abuse and provide tools to help organizations move forward. A list of publications and organizations that can provide helpful information is provided in Appendix B.

Contextual Issues

Every organization does not have to take on all strategies presented in this document. The process of implementing child sexual abuse prevention strategies takes time and will evolve differently in each organization. Not all strategies presented in this document will apply to all organizations. However, it is very important that organizations abide by their youth protection policies and procedures to avoid being criticized for not adhering to them if a youth is sexually abused. Adoption of strategies will depend on the following contextual issues:

- Organization's mission and individual activities. For example, though all youth-serving organizations are interested in helping youth develop into healthy adults, the mission of mentoring or religious organizations is often focused on fostering nurturing relationships between individual adults and youth. Because this mission results in more one-on-one activities between employees/volunteers and youth, these organizations need to adopt child sexual abuse prevention strategies that protect youth in one-on-one situations with adults.
- Culture and language of youth served by the organization.
- Insurance requirements.
- Available resources.
- State and national laws. Organizations should consult with legal representation and review state and national laws before adopting and implementing child sexual abuse prevention strategies. A good place to start is the Child Welfare Information Gateway, which provides state-specific information (www.childwelfare.gov/systemwide/laws_policies/search/index.cfm).

Balancing Caution and Caring

The same dynamics that create a nurturing environment, and may ultimately protect against child sexual abuse, can also open the doors to sexually abusive behaviors. Research has shown that youth who are emotionally insecure, needy, and unsupported may be more vulnerable to the attentions of offenders.[2] By promoting close and caring relationships between youth and adults, organizations can help youth feel supported and loved and thus reduce their risk of child sexual abuse. But that same closeness between a youth and an adult can also provide the opportunity for abuse to occur. When developing policies for child sexual abuse prevention, organizations must balance the need to keep youth safe with the need to nurture and care for them.

---

[2]Finkelhor D. Four preconditions: a model. In: Finkelhor D, editor. *Child sexual abuse: new theory and research.* New York (NY): The Free Press; 1984. p. 53–68.

Components of Child Sexual Abuse Prevention

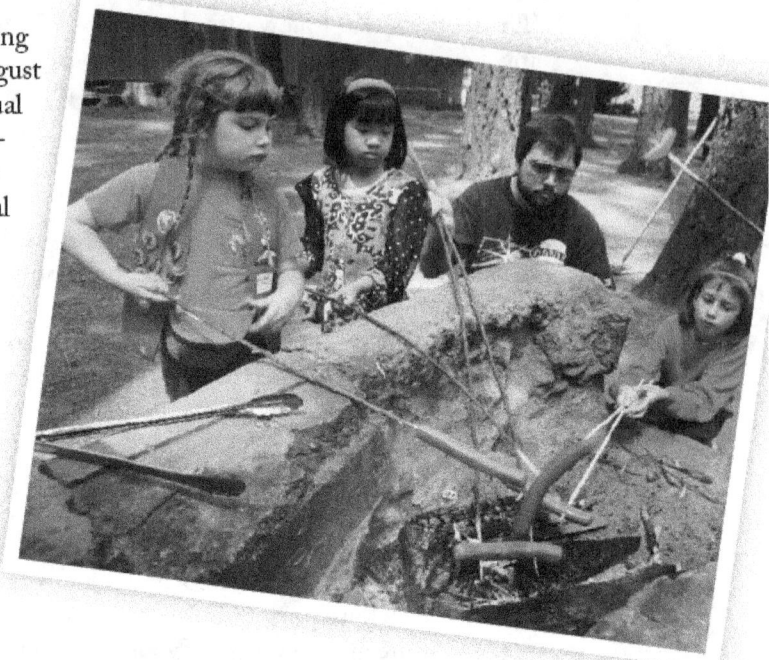

The components that follow were identified during a meeting of experts sponsored by CDC in August 2004. The experts included advocates, child sexual abuse researchers, professionals who provide prevention resources for organizations, and representatives of youth-serving organizations that have child sexual abuse prevention programs. For a list of meeting participants, see Appendix A.

Component 1:
Screening and Selecting Employees and Volunteers

Goal
To select the best possible people for staff and volunteer positions and to screen out individuals who have sexually abused youth or are at risk to abuse.

General Principles
Screening for child sexual abuse prevention should be integrated into the general screening and selection process that organizations already employ to choose the best possible candidates for positions. Child sexual abuse prevention should be one of the many areas considered when deciding whom to select. While employee/volunteer screening and selection are important, they should not be the only efforts adopted to prevent child sexual abuse.

Before you start screening
- Develop criteria that define how screening information will be used to determine an applicant's suitability.
- Identify who will make the final selection.
- Define areas of concern such as a fixation on a particular age or gender of youth or a history of crimes related to sex or violence.
- Develop consistent and systematic policies and processes for screening and selection, including a sequence and timeline for the various components of the process.
- Consult with an attorney to ensure that your screening and selection policies do not violate Title VII of the Civil Rights Act or other federal or state laws prohibiting discrimination in the workplace.

Who should be screened?
- Screen all applicants, both adults and adolescents, for all positions that will have contact with youth.
- Consider more in-depth written applications and personal interviews for adolescents, for whom work history and criminal background checks may be unavailable.
- Rigorously screen applicants who will have more autonomy as employees or volunteers.
- Do not make exceptions for people you know or have worked with in the past.

Critical Strategies for Screening and Selecting Employees and Volunteers
(These strategies are presented in roughly the order that they should be completed.)

Education about your organization and youth-protection policies
By letting applicants know your organization is serious about protecting youth, you may deter some people at risk of abusing youth from applying for staff or volunteer positions.
- Inform applicants about your organization's policies and procedures relevant to child sexual abuse prevention.
- Share your code of conduct or ethics.
- Require applicants to sign a document describing the policies and procedures of your organization to demonstrate their understanding and agreement.
- Ask applicants if they have a problem with any of the policies and procedures.

Written application

The written application provides the information you need to assess the background and interests of applicants. Questions should help you determine whether applicants have mature, adult relationships as well as clear boundaries and ethical standards for their conduct with youth. The sidebar on page 6 may help you develop appropriate questions.

- Ask about previous work and volunteer experiences.
- Ask questions pertinent to child sexual abuse screening.
- Provide a permission form for contacting personal references and performing a criminal background check. The permission statement should include an indemnification clause developed by an attorney to protect your organization from false allegations or other legal issues.
- Ask open-ended questions that encourage broad answers. These will provide material for follow-up in the personal interview and throughout the screening and selection process.
- Use disclosure statements to ask applicants about previous criminal histories of sexual offenses, violence against youth, and other criminal offenses. The applicant may not disclose past offenses, but the inquiry will demonstrate your organization's seriousness about protecting youth and potentially discourage applicants at risk for perpetrating child sexual abuse.
- Clarify that you are interested in learning about an applicant's past perpetration of child sexual abuse rather than a history of victimization.

Personal interview

The personal interview provides an opportunity to meet applicants, determine if they are a good fit for your organization, and ask additional questions to screen for child sexual abuse risk factors. The sidebar on page 6 may help you develop interview questions.

- Ask open-ended questions that encourage discussion.
- Clarify and expand upon the applicant's answers to questions from the written application.

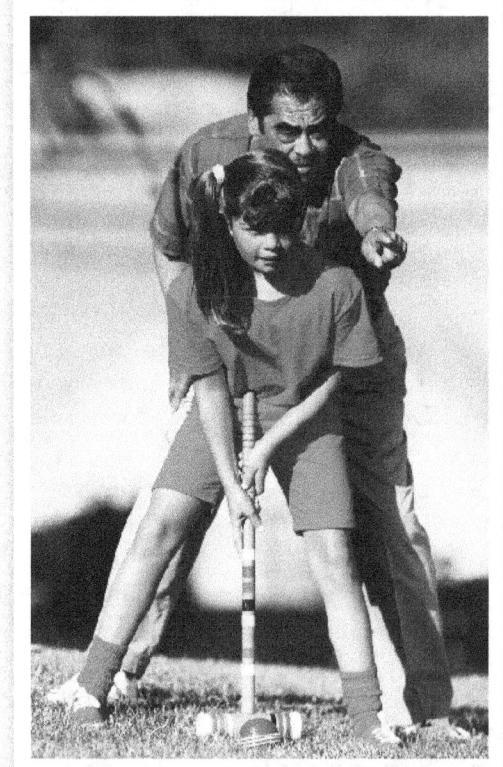

The following questions may be used in a written application or personal interview. A single answer should not determine whether an applicant is selected or rejected. Along with other forms of information, answers to these questions can help you build a more complete picture of an applicant. Additional questions may be found in various publications and policies in the "Resource List and Sample Policies" section. (See Appendix B.)

- *What type of supervisory situation do you prefer?*
  If applicants are very independent, they may not fit in an organization whose policies and procedures require close supervision.

- *What age/sex of youth do you want to work with? How would you feel about working with a different age/sex?*
  If an applicant seems fixated on one age/sex, be wary. However, it may be that the applicant has experience or is gifted with working with certain age groups. Asking follow-up questions about why an applicant has a strong preference can help you determine if there is cause for concern.

- *Is there anyone who might suggest that you should not work with youth? Why or why not?*

- *Why do you want the job?*

- *What would you do in a particular situation?*
  Set up scenarios that involve potential concerns, boundary issues, or youth protection policies and interactions to gauge the applicant's response. Be concerned if applicants disregard the organization's policies and procedures or handle a situation poorly.

- *What makes you a good candidate for working with youth? What would your friends or colleagues say about how you interact with youth?*

- *What other hobbies or activities do you enjoy?*
  Determine if applicants have mature, adult relationships—not just relationships with youth.

Reference checks

Reference checks provide additional information about applicants and help verify previous work and volunteer history.

- Obtain verbal—not just written—references for applicants. Conversations can elicit much more information than written responses.
- Match references with employment and volunteer history. Is anyone important missing from the references, such as the supervisor from the applicant's most recent job? To provide a more complete picture of the applicant, the references should come from a variety of sources and should not be limited to family members or friends.
- Be aware that many employers will only provide basic information, such as dates of employment or rehiring eligibility. If a former employer will only provide limited information, clarify whether the person providing the reference is limiting information because of company policy.

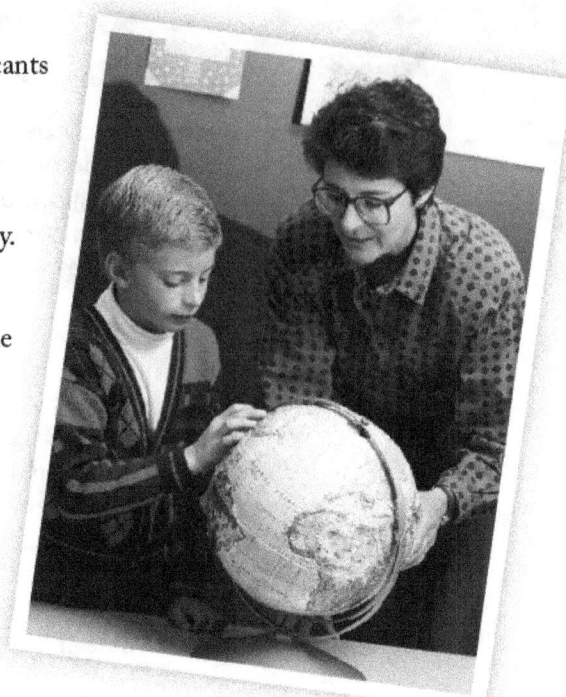

The following questions may be useful for reference checks:

- How would you describe the personal characteristics of the applicant?
- How does the applicant interact with youth?
- Why would this person be a good candidate for working with youth? Is there any reason this person should not work with youth?
- Have you seen the applicant discipline youth (other than his or her own children)?
- Would you hire this person again? Would you want him or her in your organization in the future?

Criminal background checks

Criminal background checks are an important tool in screening and selection. However, they have limitations. Criminal background checks will not identify most sexual offenders because most have not been caught. When this report was published, an efficient, effective, and affordable national background screening system was not available.

- Use background checks as one part of child sexual abuse prevention efforts. Using background checks alone may give your organization a false sense of security.
- Save time and resources by delaying criminal background checks until the end of the screening and selection process. Applicants who do not make it through the written applications, personal interviews, and reference checks will not need a criminal background check.
- Obtain permission from applicants before beginning a criminal background check.
- Determine the type and level of check required for each applicant. Types of checks include name, fingerprint, sex offender registries, and social security number. Checks may be implemented at county, state, and national levels. Records are not always linked or comprehensive, so a thorough search may be needed to address concerns about an applicant. For example, if an applicant has moved frequently, checks in multiple states may be necessary.
- Plan for the time and financial resources needed to conduct background checks.
- Decide which offenses to examine in the background checks and which offenses will disqualify applicants. For child sexual abuse, absolute disqualifiers include violent behavior and

child sexual abuse perpetration history. Depending on the risk of the situation or the mission of your organization, drug and driving offenses may also be disqualifiers. Arrest data are not grounds for disqualification; only offenses resulting in convictions may be used.

- Develop procedures to keep the results of criminal background checks confidential. Select a secure storage location and limit access to the files.
- Ensure that your organization's process for conducting criminal background checks is legally sound. Consult county, state, and national laws and regulations, as well as your organization's attorney and insurance company, as needed.

Additional Strategies to Consider

Assessment of home environment

The need for assessing an applicant's home environment depends on the mission of your organization. This may be an essential strategy for mentoring programs where youth meet with mentors at their homes, but it may be irrelevant and inappropriate for other organizations, such as sleep-away camps or after-school programs.

Checking applicants against internal records

This strategy involves keeping lists of applicants who are disqualified during the screening process and employees/volunteers who are dismissed because of an offense. During the screening and selection process, your organization would then check current applicants against these lists to make sure the applicant has not been previously disqualified or dismissed.

Internet search

Some organizations may choose to search the internet to find additional relevant information about an applicant. Be aware that more than one person can share the same name and that it may be difficult to verify the accuracy of information found on the internet.

Component 2:
Guidelines on Interactions Between Individuals

Goal

To ensure the safety of youth in their interactions with employees/volunteers and with each other.

General Principles

Guidelines on interactions between individuals should be determined by an organization's mission and activities. For example, organizations that promote one-on-one activities between adults and youth may need different interaction guidelines than programs built around group activities. Organizations should develop interaction policies before situations arise. The strategies listed below should be tailored to the developmental age and maturity of the youth and employees/volunteers. Strategies should also match the cultural context of the population served by the organization. In this section, "adult" refers to any individual in a supervisory position, including youth.

Balancing positive and negative

*   Find a balance between encouraging positive and appropriate interactions and discouraging inappropriate and harmful interactions.
*   Adopt strategies with this balance in mind to ensure that youth benefit from your program without risk of sexual abuse or harm.

Critical Strategies for Guidelines on Interactions between Individuals
Appropriate/inappropriate/harmful behaviors

Appropriate, positive interactions among youth and between employees/volunteers and youth are essential in supporting positive youth development, making youth feel valued, and providing the caring connections that serve as protective factors for youth. Conversely, inappropriate or harmful interactions put youth at risk for adverse physical and emotional outcomes. Organizations should identify behaviors that fall into the categories of appropriate, inappropriate, and harmful. These categorizations can be spelled out in your code of conduct or ethics. Carefully balance the benefits of appropriate interactions with the risks associated with inappropriate interactions. See page 10 for examples of appropriate/innappropriate/harmful behaviors.

Ratios of employees/volunteers to youth

The goal of setting ratios for the numbers of employees/volunteers to youth is to ensure the safety of the youth. There is no standard ratio for all situations. When making decisions about ratios, consider contextual variables such as:

*   Age and developmental level of youth and employees/volunteers. If youth or employees/volunteers are young, you may need a lower ratio, that is, fewer youth per adult.
*   Risk of the activity. Does it involve a great deal of isolation from others?
*   Location of the activity. Is it in a classroom that is easy to monitor or at a park, where it is easier to lose track of individuals?

Encourage employees/volunteers to actively interact with the youth to maintain adequate supervision and monitoring. Even with a satisfactory ratio of employees/volunteers to youth, the youth are not being monitored if all of the employees/volunteers are immersed in their own conversations in a corner of the room.

Examples of Appropriate/Inappropriate/Harmful Behavior from Youth-serving Organizations

Sometimes it is unclear if a behavior is appropriate, inappropriate, or harmful. For example, intimate contact, such as kissing, may be developmentally appropriate for older youth, but may be inappropriate within the confines of the organization. It may even be harmful if the kissing is coercive. Another example involves hugging. Hugging may be appropriate and positive in some circumstances, but it can also be inappropriate if the child is not receptive, if the employee/volunteer is hugging too often or for too long, or if the contact is romanticized or sexually intimate.

Verbal communication
Appropriate:
- Praise
- Positive reinforcement for good work/behavior

Inappropriate/harmful:
- Sexually provocative or degrading comments
- Risqué jokes

Physical behavior
Appropriate:
- Pats on the back or shoulder

Inappropriate/harmful:
- Patting the buttocks
- Intimate/romantic/sexual contact
- Corporal punishment
- Showing pornography or involving youth in pornographic activities

One-on-one interactions

Some organizations have a policy to limit one-on-one interactions between youth and adults (i.e., having at least two adults present at all times with youth). The goal of such a policy is to prevent the isolation of one adult and one youth, a situation that elevates the risk for child sexual abuse. This strategy must be modified based on the mission of your organization.

- Limit one-on-one interactions whenever possible by having at least two adults present at all times with youth.
- Choose one of three options relating to this policy:
    - Make this a mandatory policy at all times.
    - Make this policy dependent on the risk of the activity or situation, such as overnight trips.
    - Maintain other safeguards such as extra supervision or contact with youth and employees/volunteers and more stringent screening if the mission of your organization requires one-on-one time between employees/volunteers and youth (e.g., mentoring programs).

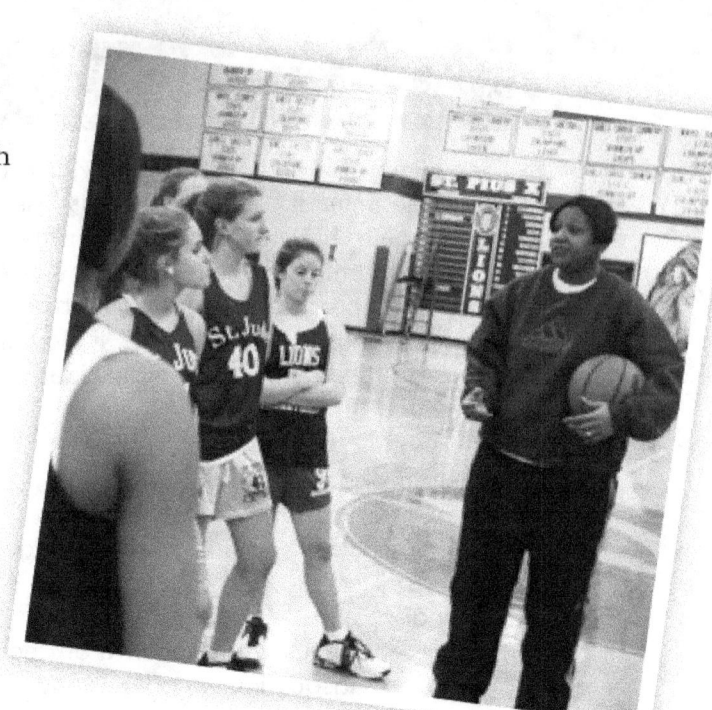

Risk of interactions between youth

Your organization needs to address interactions among youth in addition to monitoring interactions between employees/volunteers and youth. Many strategies that focus on the interactions between employees/volunteers and youth can be tailored to address interactions among youth.

- Address all situations where unsupervised youth can sexually or physically abuse other youth. For example, if your organization has a policy that prevents adults from being present in locker rooms because of the risk of child sexual abuse, this may result in a situation where unsupervised youth can sexually or physically abuse other youth. A potential solution is adopting a policy that requires more than one adult to be present at all times.
- Develop policies to deal with bullying and sexual abuse so that positive interactions can be promoted while acknowledging that some interactions are inappropriate or harmful.

Prohibitions and restrictions on certain activities

Some activities, such as hazing and secret ceremonies, overnight trips, bathing, changing, bathroom interactions, and nighttime activities, pose greater risks for child sexual abuse. Prohibiting or restricting such activities will depend largely on the context of your organization. For example, a sleep-away camp would not be able to prohibit overnight trips or bathing.

Out-of-program contact restrictions

There are two types of out-of-program contact restrictions. The first type involves the contact of youth with employees/volunteers outside the context of the program. Your organization should limit contact between employees/volunteers and youth to organization-sanctioned activities and programs and/or to certain locations, such as activities within your organization's building.

The second type is contact between youth and people not affiliated with your organization that occurs while youth are under the care of your organization.

- Develop a system for monitoring the comings and goings of all youth and adults who enter and leave your facility. This system might include procedures for signing in and out.
- Develop specific policies about interactions between youth and people not affiliated with your organization if it is located in a building that houses more than just your program or if your organization's activities take place in public areas (e.g., sports field).

Caregiver information and permission

Your organization should obtain addresses and contact information for youth and caregivers (i.e., parents and guardians). This information should never be released to unauthorized individuals. Your organization also should obtain permission from caregivers for youth to participate in certain activities, such as field trips, late-night activities, and overnight trips.

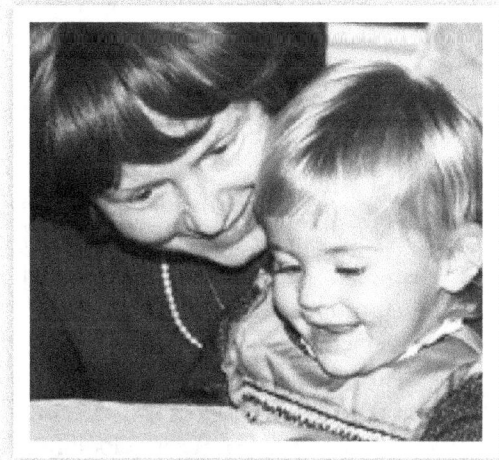

- Inform caregivers about what their children/ youth will be doing and where they will be going.
- Allow caregivers to have input on what activities or interactions they are comfortable with for their children.

Responsibility for youth

Your organization should clarify when it is responsible for youth and when caregivers are responsible.

- Develop a policy on when your organization starts and stops being responsible for youth.
- Consider who is responsible for youth before and after activities officially begin.
- Communicate the policy to caregivers and youth in writing. Organizations may also want caregivers to sign an acknowledgement that they have read and understand the policy.

Additional Strategies to Consider

Other ways to control interactions between individuals

Identify ways to monitor interactions, such as instituting a buddy system to prevent isolation of youth with employees/volunteers.

Component 3:
Monitoring Behavior

Goal
To prevent, recognize, and respond to inappropriate and harmful behaviors and to reinforce appropriate behaviors.

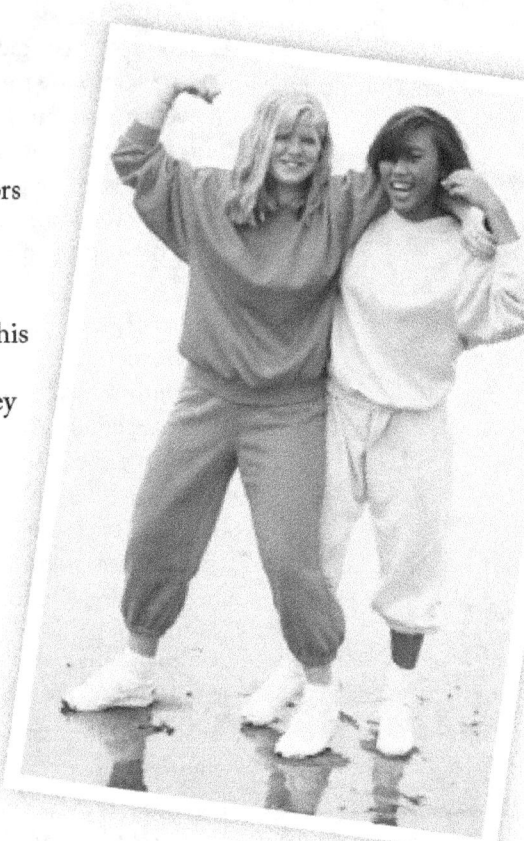

General Principles
Monitoring involves observing interactions and reacting appropriately. This includes both employee/volunteer–youth and youth-youth interactions. Youth leaders often require more supervision and monitoring because they are young, may lack judgment, and are harder to screen. Define areas for monitoring based on the organization's mission and activities.

Monitor inappropriate or harmful behaviors
- Refer to your organization's interaction policies and what has been defined as inappropriate or harmful behavior. (See "Appropriate/ Innappropriate/Harmful Behaviors" on pages 9 and 10.)
- Understand the boundaries that your organization has established and identify when someone has crossed the line. Potential inappropriate behaviors include employees/volunteers showing favoritism, giving gifts, and looking for time alone with youth.

Monitor potential risk situations
Acknowledge that some situations pose more risk for inappropriate or harmful behavior than others. For example, interactions during an overnight trip are harder to monitor than interactions in a classroom.

Monitor appropriate behaviors
- Acknowledge, praise, and encourage appropriate behaviors.
- Reward and reinforce positive interactions between employees/volunteers and youth.

Critical Strategies for Monitoring Behavior
Responding to what is observed
Your organization must be prepared to respond to interactions among youth and between employees/volunteers and youth.
- Develop a monitoring protocol so that employees/volunteers are clear about their roles and responsibilities. Employees/volunteers should be prepared to respond immediately to inappropriate or harmful behavior, potential risk situations, and potential boundary violations.
- Enforce the protocol so that appropriate actions follow. Supervisors need to redirect inappropriate behaviors to promote positive behaviors, confront inappropriate or harmful behaviors, and report these behaviors if necessary. (For more information on reporting, see "Responding to Inappropriate Behavior, Breaches in Policy, and Allegations or Suspicions of Child Sexual Abuse" on page 17.)

Roles and responsibilities
All employees/volunteers should be responsible for monitoring behavior and interactions within your organization. Everyone needs to know how and what to monitor. Define roles and responsibilities

by including monitoring within a job description, specifying what employees/volunteers need to do from the very beginning, and providing training.

Clear reporting structure within organization
Your organization should have a well-defined reporting structure so people know who to contact if they observe potentially inappropriate or harmful behavior.
- Require employees/volunteers to report any behaviors and practices that may be harmful.
- Establish direct-line and back-up reporting systems within your organization. The back-up option should be used if the incident involves the direct-line authority.
- Create a climate that encourages people to question confusing or uncertain behaviors and practices.

Observation and contact with employees/volunteers
Your organization should use multiple monitoring methods to get a clear picture of how individuals are interacting.
- Use formal supervision, including regular evaluations.
- Use informal supervision, including regular and random observation (e.g., roving and checking interactions throughout an activity period), and maintain frequent contact with employees/volunteers and youth who interact off-site.

Documentation that monitoring has occurred
Although it may be clear when other child sexual abuse prevention strategies, such as screening or environmental policies, have been implemented in your organization, it is harder to be sure that adequate monitoring is occurring. Documenting that monitoring has occurred emphasizes to employees/volunteers that it is an essential, nonnegotiable part of your organization's child sexual abuse prevention efforts.
- Use written records.
- Provide positive reinforcement when good supervision occurs.

Component 4:
Ensuring Safe Environments

Goal
To keep youth from situations in which they are at increased risk for sexual abuse.

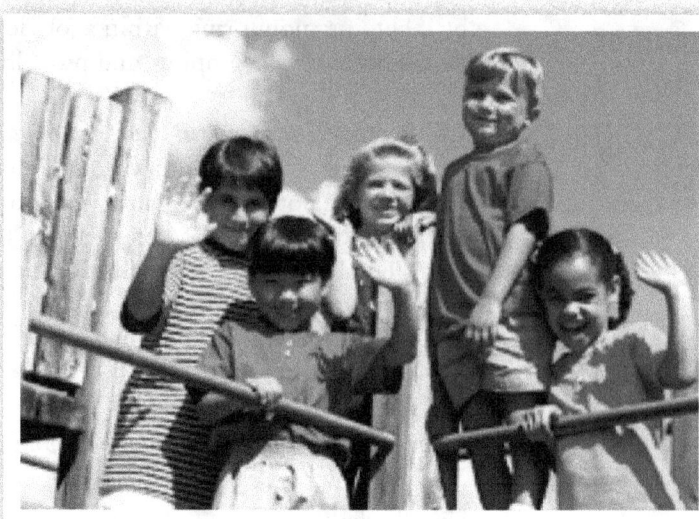

General Principles
Environmental strategies will vary depending on the organization. Strategies will be different for organizations with physical sites (e.g., a day care, school), organizations with multiple sites for activities (e.g., some sports and recreation organizations), and organizations with leased or undefined space (e.g., mentoring organizations). The risk of the environment should be considered regardless of an organization's physical space. If an organization does not control its own space, back-up strategies should be used to ensure youth and employees/volunteers can be monitored.

Critical Strategies for Ensuring Safe Environments
Visibility
Building or choosing spaces that are open and visible to multiple people can create an environment where individuals at risk for sexually abusive behaviors do not feel comfortable abusing.

Use the following methods to increase visibility:
- Landscape to ensure open visible spaces with no possible concealment.
- Have clear lines of sight throughout the building.
- Secure areas not used for program purposes to prevent youth from being isolated (e.g., lock closets and storerooms).
- Install windows in doors.
- Institute a "no closed door" policy.
- Install bright lighting in all areas.

Privacy when toileting, showering, changing clothes
Your organization should develop policies and procedures for reducing risk during activities such as toileting, showering, and changing clothes that consider not just the risk of employee/volunteer sexual abuse, but also the risk of inappropriate or harmful contact among youth.

Access control
Your organization should monitor who is present at all times.
- Develop policies and procedures for admitting and releasing youth so their whereabouts are always known.
- Have policies and procedures for monitoring which people outside of your organization are allowed in and under what circumstances.

Off-site activity guidelines

Your organization should define and communicate its on-site and off-site physical boundaries.

- Decide and communicate when and where your organization is responsible for the youth it serves. This is particularly important in a multi-organization facility and on field trips.
- Develop environmental policies for field trips and other off-site activities, such as how to handle off-site bathroom breaks and use of public transportation.

Transportation policies

Your organization should define who is responsible for transporting youth to and from regular activities and special events (e.g., field trips, overnight trips).

Decide how to answer the following questions:

- When is your organization responsible for transportation?
- When are caregivers responsible?
- Can a youth ride in a car with an employee/volunteer? If yes, under what circumstances? For example, can a youth be alone with an employee/volunteer in a car?
- What are pick-up procedures at the end of the day or the event?

Additional Strategies to Consider

Territoriality

The goal of this strategy is to visually send a message that the program is unified, cohesive, and not permeable to threats. Some examples of this strategy include making navigation easy with signage and overstating the appearance of staff with uniforms or similar clothing.

Monitoring devices (e.g., video cameras)

This strategy implies that there is an infrastructure or staff behind the monitoring devices. If you install these devices, be sure to provide the infrastructure to uphold that implicit promise.

Component 5:
Responding to Inappropriate Behavior, Breaches in Policy, and Allegations and Suspicions of Child Sexual Abuse

Goal
To respond quickly and appropriately to (1) inappropriate or harmful behavior, (2) infractions of child sexual abuse prevention policies, and (3) evidence or allegations of child sexual abuse.

General Principles
The ultimate aim of child sexual abuse prevention efforts within youth-serving organizations is to prevent child sexual abuse from ever occurring; however, an organization needs to have communicated clearly what it and its employees/volunteers should do if policies are violated or if child sexual abuse occurs.

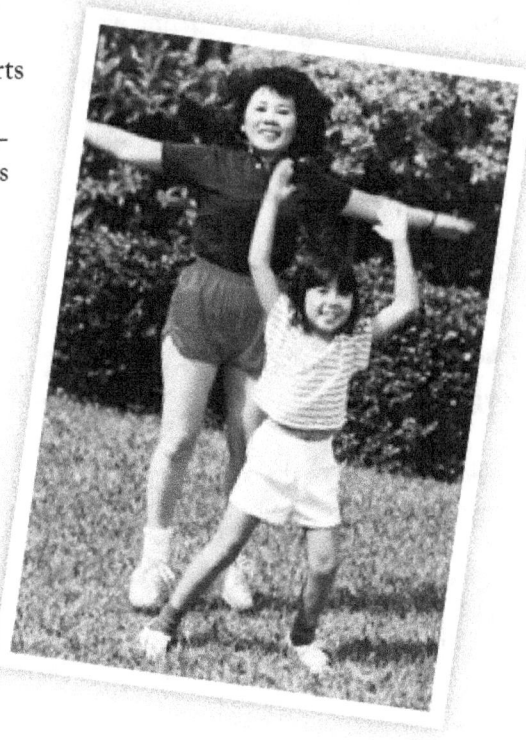

Define inappropriate and appropriate strategies
- Clarify that it is not the role of an employee/volunteer or your organization to evaluate or investigate an allegation or suspicion.
- Let child protective services, law enforcement, and child advocacy centers investigate allegations or suspicions.
- Know that an organization's investigation can harm the youth or the legal investigative process.

Partnering with others
- Work with a lawyer to develop a reporting policy to ensure that it is appropriate and legal.
- Partner with child protective services, law enforcement, and child advocacy centers (www.nca-online.org) before any allegations arise to form relationships and ensure that policies are in line with the law.

Critical Strategies for Responding to Inappropriate Behavior, Breaches in Policy, and Allegations and Suspicions of Child Sexual Abuse
What to respond to within the organization and what to report to the authorities
As discussed previously, it is often difficult to find the balance between being vigilant and protective of youth and being so hyper-vigilant that the positive parts of programs (e.g., relationships between adults and youth) are lost. In responding, the need for this balance involves recognizing the tension between over-reacting and under-reacting. By developing policies before any inappropriate behavior occurs, your organization can set reasonable expectations for responding.
- Define the continuum of appropriate, inappropriate, and harmful behavior.
- Delineate what behaviors your organization will respond to internally and what behaviors will require reporting to the authorities. For example, if a youth tells a sexually risqué joke, your organization may inform a direct-line supervisor and/or the youth's caregiver; provide the youth with guidance, redirection, and instruction; and/or file an incident report. However, if a youth or employee/volunteer forces sexual contact with a youth, this violation should always be reported to the appropriate authorities in accord with the procedures outlined in your policy.

- Act on infractions of your organization's child sexual abuse prevention policy. If an employee/volunteer has breached a policy, such as having contact with youth outside of your organization, your organization must take action, even when child sexual abuse is not suspected. The consequences of violating policies should be explicit and violations should be addressed immediately. However, if abuse is suspected, it should be reported to authorities immediately.
- Report when an employee/volunteer witnesses or learns about sexual abuse of youth by any of the following individuals:
  - Volunteer/employee.
  - Another youth within the organization.
  - Someone outside of the organization (e.g., caregiver).
- Tailor strategies and policies to each type of child sexual abuse. For example, identify to whom reports are made. In most states, child protective services is responsible for caretaker abuse, and law enforcement is responsible for abuse by all other individuals. Responsibility can vary by state, so consult experts such as those in your nearest child advocacy center, your state sexual violence coalition, or your local rape crisis center in order to incorporate state guidelines into your policies.

Reporting process

If evidence of child sexual abuse has surfaced or an allegation has been made, a formal report needs to be made to an outside agency. Ensure that your organization's reporting policies are consistent with current state law. The following strategies address policies related to reporting evidence or allegations of child sexual abuse to outside agencies.

- Who must report
  - Mandatory reporters (i.e., those individuals required by the state to report suspicions of child abuse and neglect to the authorities). To research laws about mandatory reporters in your state, go to www.childwelfare.gov/systemwide/laws_policies/search/index.cfm.
  - Employees/volunteers if they are state-designated mandatory reporters or if your organization requires that they report suspicions of child abuse and neglect.

- To whom to report
  - Have clear guidelines about how and when to report allegations and suspicions to authorities. Allegations and suspicions should be reported to very few people inside the organization before authorities are contacted to expedite the process and minimize the number of times a youth has to repeat allegations.
  - Be explicit that the head of your organization is professionally and legally accountable for ensuring that all cases of abuse are reported to the proper authorities.
  - Delineate which external authorities (i.e., child protective services or law enforcement) should be contacted in different types of abuse cases. Consult state guidelines to ensure your policies are consistent with them.

- When to report
  - Report to the authorities any time there is a reasonable suspicion of child abuse or neglect.
    - Consult child protective services, law enforcement, or a child advocacy center to ensure your organization is defining reasonable suspicion appropriately according to your state guidelines.
    - Obtain the help of a child advocacy center in deciding if reporting an allegation is appropriate because these centers work with law enforcement, social workers, lawyers, and mental health professionals. More information on these organizations is available in the "Resource List and Sample Policies" section. (See Appendix B.)
    - Do not conduct your own investigation, but depending on the circumstances, it may be appropriate to ask a few clarifying questions of the youth or the person making the allegation to adequately report the suspicion or allegation to the authorities. For example, in one case, a young girl said, "My daddy put his thing in my mouth and it hurt." When asked what she meant, the youth replied that her father had stuck his fingers too far into her mouth when attempting to get out a loose tooth. The person who was speaking with the girl at first thought that a report needed to be made, but then slowed down to clarify what had occurred. After doing so, it was clear no report was needed.

Internal records

Although your organization should not investigate allegations or suspicions of child sexual abuse in lieu of reporting them to the authorities, it should develop a system to track allegations and suspicions of child sexual abuse cases.

- Include child sexual abuse as a category on general incident reporting forms for significant physical injuries. These forms should be completed by employees/volunteers who first learn of the abuse through hearing an allegation or making an observation.
- Review the general incident reporting forms. This step should be carried out by the supervisor of the employee/volunteer.
- Refer child sexual abuse reports to a higher-level individual, preferably a trained internal or hired investigator, for the purpose of reviewing your organization's procedures. This individual should do an incident review after each allegation to determine what went wrong and how a similar scenario can be prevented in the future. For example, was a policy or a step in a policy not followed? How can policies be modified to prevent another occurrence?
- Record the resolutions of child sexual abuse cases.

Confidentiality policy

Because of the sensitive nature of child sexual abuse cases, your organization should decide in advance what information should remain private and what information can be made public.

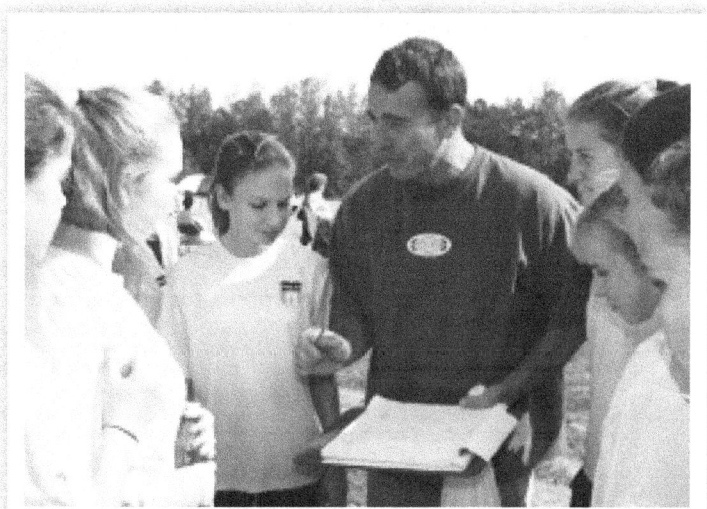

- Withhold the names of potential victims, the accused perpetrator, and the people who made the report to the authorities.
- Decide whether to inform the community that an allegation has been made.
- Ensure that your organization's confidentiality policy is consistent with state legal requirements.

Response to the press and the community

Your organization should decide on a strategy for responding to the press and the community before an allegation has been made.

- Designate a spokesperson for questions and inquiries.
- Have employees/volunteers go through training on how to deal with the press and the community, if appropriate.

Membership/employment of alleged offenders

Remember that an allegation of child sexual abuse does not equate to guilt. The person alleged to have engaged in sexually abusive behavior should not be labeled as an offender or sexual abuser. However, once a suspicion or allegation has been communicated, it needs to be reported to the authorities, and your organization must take certain steps to protect the youth under its care. A decision must be made whether to suspend membership or employment.

- Suspend membership or employment immediately after reporting the child sexual abuse or put the alleged offender on probation until the case is resolved legally. Have an appeal process in which people found not guilty of perpetration in court may apply to return to their former positions in the organization.
- Develop policies on how to deal appropriately and responsibly with alleged or convicted offenders if your organization decides that it may not be appropriate to revoke membership or employment. Some organizations, particularly faith-based ones or those dealing with youth-on-youth sexual abuse, may decide that revoking membership sends the wrong message. Because these organizations need to manage circumstances in which alleged victims and offenders may be together, a well-constructed policy can help deal with this difficult situation.
  - Require limited access agreements in which alleged or convicted offenders can attend a worship service or activity that does not involve youth but may not be involved in any activities specific to youth. These individuals may also be required to attend permitted services and activities with a "buddy" or another adult who has agreed to stay with them at all times.

- Require informed supervision. Make sure at least one staff member is informed of the sexual abuse and is instructed to supervise vigilantly the accused adult or youth in his or her interaction with the program and/or organization.
- Employ restorative practices. (See "Additional Strategies to Consider" below.)

Additional Strategies to Consider
Support for victims and families
Organizations may want to provide support for victims and their families to help them cope with the sexual abuse.
- Provide referrals for victims and their families to child sexual abuse organizations and counselors or therapists.
- Reimburse victims and families for counseling.
- Offer restorative justice approaches. Restorative practices are a way to have a respectful and safe dialogue when a misunderstanding or a harm has occurred. If your organization is interested in using restorative justice, seek assistance from organizations with expertise in these techniques and refer to the "Resource List and Sample Policies" section. (See Appendix B.)

Coping process for the organization and community
The organization and community as a whole may need help getting past the child sexual abuse that has occurred.
- Adopt strategies such as showing that steps are being taken to deal appropriately with the situation, providing support groups, and having forums to discuss the topic and answer questions.
- Adopt a policy for notifying the wider organization and caregivers that child sexual abuse has happened. But before doing so, determine what information is appropriate to share. (See "Confidentiality Policy" on page 20.)
- Train caregivers on how to talk to youth about child sexual abuse.
- Debrief or offer support and counseling for reporters and bystanders.
- Seek assistance in using restorative justice approaches to help the community heal.

Component 6:
Training about Child Sexual Abuse Prevention

Goal
To give people information and skills to help them prevent and respond to child sexual abuse.

This section will first present general training guidelines and will then cover specific information on education and training for three types of people related to organizations: employees/volunteers, caregivers, and youth.

General Principles
To ensure that child sexual abuse training is effective and fits with other strategies, organizations should follow several guidelines.

Goals in training
- Set measurable goals. What are the desired behaviors or performance changes in trainees? What is essential that people gain from the training?
- Plan the training to meet goals.
- Evaluate the training periodically to ensure that it meets goals.
- Decide if your organization wants to use an overarching frame. Two that have been used in other organizations are (1) healthy sexuality and (2) rights and responsibilities. The healthy sexuality frame for child sexual abuse education helps individuals distinguish child sexual abuse from something that is healthy and normal. The rights and responsibilities frame involves teaching individuals that they have the right to be treated appropriately and the responsibility to treat others appropriately.

Integration of content into the entire organization
- Ensure that training content is modeled by everyone in your organization, from management to employees/volunteers.
- Training content should be evident in performance measures, supervisors' feedback to employees/volunteers, caregivers' observations, and treatment of youth by your organization.
- Meld elements of your organization's philosophy or mission with the child sexual abuse training. For example, a faith-based organization may want to incorporate elements of its faith into the training content.

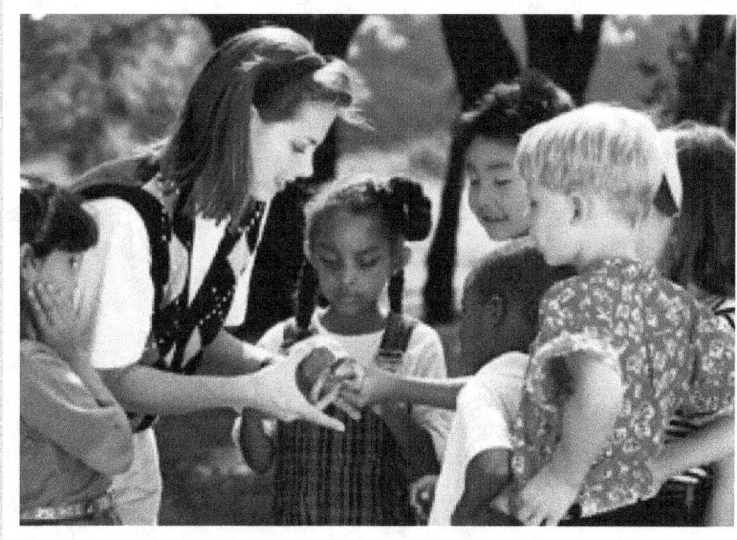

Training Techniques

There are many ways to provide information and teach skills to individuals. Delivery mechanisms, level of interactivity, frequency, and training methods all need to be considered when designing a training or education program.

Delivery mechanisms

Delivery mechanisms can use a great deal of technology or none at all. Training messages, numbers of trainees, resources, flexibility, and integration with other training within the organization should be considered when choosing a delivery mechanism. Be sensitive to dealing with the emotional topic of child sexual abuse in impersonal formats (e.g., online, videos, CDs).

- Online. Interaction is key to making sure that people learn the material, so using interactive online techniques may work better than passive ones.
- Videos/CDs.
- In person.
- Written.
- Combinations of delivery mechanisms (e.g., some online, some in person).

Interactivity

Training can be passive, interactive, or somewhere in between.

- Use passive training, in which trainees do not interact with anyone else (e.g., video), for raising awareness.
- Use interactive training, in which trainees interact with the trainer and/or other trainees, for skills building.

Frequency

Your organization needs to reinforce the content of child sexual abuse training.

- Ensure that training is ongoing and not just a one-time event.
- Educate in both formal training sessions and in informal settings, such as conversations.

Methods

Using several methods to train individuals on child sexual abuse reinforces messages and allows individuals with different learning styles to absorb information and skills.

- Present case studies to elicit discussion and suggestions for handling situations and walking through problem-solving.
- Ask people to role play situations.
- Use journaling.
- Have outside professionals conduct training; this may emphasize the importance of the topic.

Mechanisms to ensure that training happens

Because training can be expensive and time-consuming, mechanisms must be in place to ensure that training is conducted.

- For organizations: develop a regular training schedule or repeat trainings when a specified number of new employees/volunteers have been hired. In addition, integrate training into the overall child sexual abuse prevention policy and into some staff member's work plans.
- For individuals: require periodic certification based on training completion.
- To save time, money, and resources, your organization can do the following:
  - Ask for help from groups who have already done this type of training.
  - Work together with a group of similar organizations to develop and implement training.
  - Partner with other organizations, including child advocacy centers, sexual violence coalitions, and universities.

Creation of a safe space

Create an environment in which trainees feel comfortable raising questions and concerns. Being receptive to questions reduces barriers to coming forward, reporting, and being proactive about preventing and responding to child sexual abuse.

Point of contact for child sexual abuse

- Designate one point of contact for questions and concerns to ensure messages about child sexual abuse are communicated consistently. This point of contact can be one individual or a group within a division of your organization.
- State explicitly that every employee/volunteer is still responsible for preventing and responding to child sexual abuse.

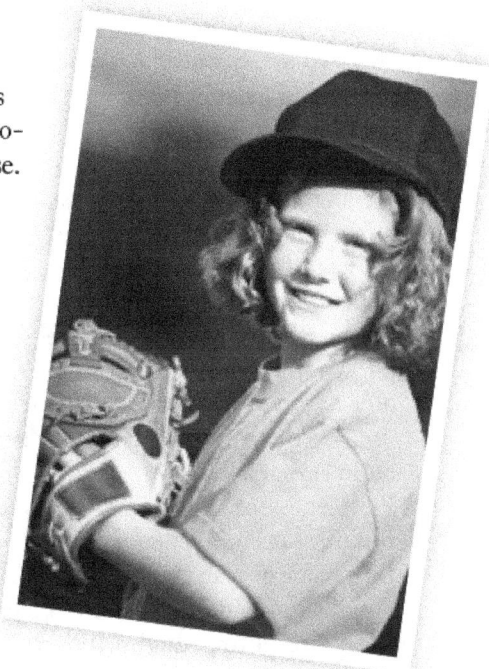

Training Employees/Volunteers

Who needs training?

The following employees/volunteers should be trained in child sexual abuse prevention:

- People with access to or supervision over youth, including adults and youth in leadership positions.
- People responsible for enforcing child sexual abuse policies or overseeing people in the chain of command (e.g., supervisors of employees/volunteers with access to or control over youth).
- Management and leaders in your organization, even those without contact with youth, so concepts can be reinforced throughout the culture of your organization.
- New and current employees/volunteers.

Differences between employees and volunteers

Depending on the organization, education/training for employees and volunteers may differ. For example, employees and volunteers may need varied curricula in a mentoring organization, whereas an after-school program may choose to educate employees and volunteers together.

Critical Content for Training Employees/Volunteers

All policies and procedures organization chooses

Employees/volunteers should be trained on all of the policies and procedures discussed in this document that your organization chooses to adopt.

Child sexual abuse information

To prevent child sexual abuse, employees/volunteers need to understand general information about child sexual abuse (e.g., what child sexual abuse is, how often it occurs).

- Provide a definition of child sexual abuse.
- Define the continuum of appropriate, inappropriate, and harmful behavior from your organization's perspective.
- Provide information about the prevalence of child sexual abuse.
- Describe risk and protective factors for victimization and perpetration.
- Address common myths about offenders, such as the myth that most people who sexually abuse are strangers to the youth.

Importance of preventing child sexual abuse

Employees/volunteers need to understand why they should be concerned with preventing child sexual abuse.

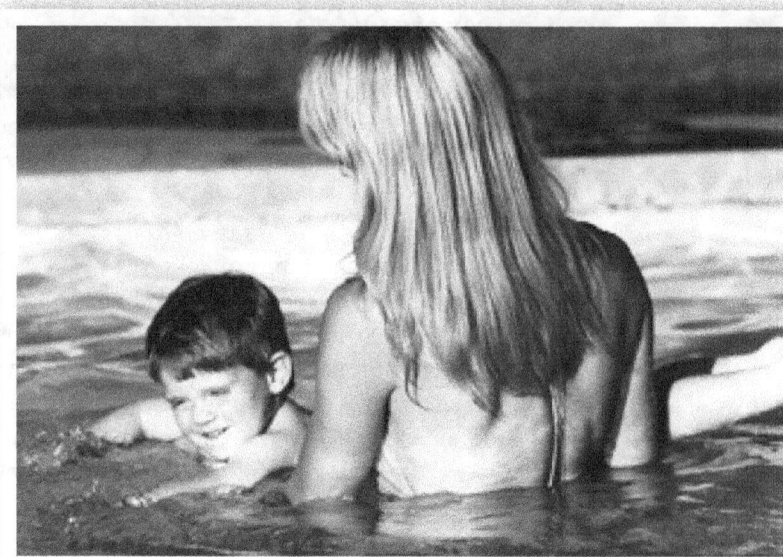

- Emphasize that employees/volunteers are an integral part of your organization's efforts to create a safe, healthy, and respectful environment.
- Explain that child sexual abuse policies protect youth from sexual abuse, adults and youth from allegations of sexual abuse, and organizations from being accused of not doing enough to prevent child sexual abuse.
- Help employees/volunteers feel comfortable and motivated to prevent child sexual abuse. For example, provide employees/volunteers with information about preventing child sexual abuse and opportunities to practice how to handle situations (e.g., monitoring interactions).
- Give employees/volunteers opportunities to ask questions and express concerns about child sexual abuse prevention.

Personal conduct

In addition to training on the elements of child sexual abuse prevention related to interactions between individuals, your organization may want to train employees/volunteers on how to conduct themselves with youth and with other employees/volunteers.

- Define appropriate conduct.
- Describe how to deal appropriately with risky or compromising situations, such as romantic crushes of youth on employees/volunteers or of employees/volunteers on youth.
- Acknowledge the power differential between adults and youth and between youth leaders and youth.
- Inform employees/volunteers of their responsibility to act when they see or hear about inappropriate or harmful behavior.

Healthy development of youth

Employees/volunteers should learn about healthy youth development so they can (1) promote positive development in the areas of self-confidence, independence, and social interactivity and (2) understand and be aware of risk behaviors in which youth may engage.

- Teach employees/volunteers about healthy youth development and when certain behaviors are appropriate.
- Educate employees/volunteers about sexual development and how to distinguish between healthy and inappropriate or harmful behaviors when monitoring interactions.
- Keep in mind that some behavior that is considered developmentally appropriate may create problems for organizations when it is done at inappropriate times.

Protective factors

Employees/volunteers should know that youth-serving organizations exist in order to provide a healthy and safe environment where youth can thrive. The very things that youth-serving organizations do may be protective against child sexual abuse. For example, close, caring, and connected relationships between youth and employees/volunteers can be extremely beneficial for youth development and can help youth feel supported and loved. This may protect youth from child sexual abuse. Because of the nature of the interactions in these relationships, however, they can also put youth at risk of being sexually abused by employees/volunteers.

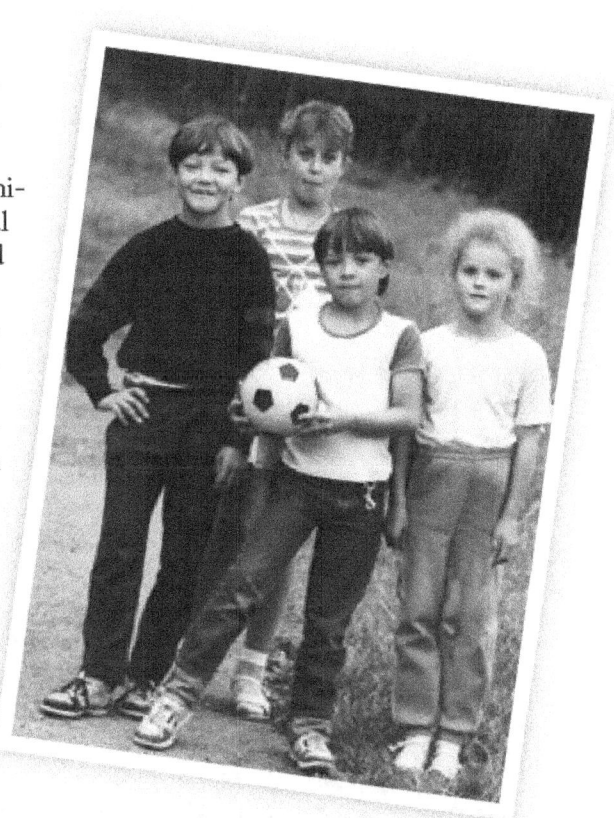

- Help employees/volunteers learn to maintain a balance between providing a nurturing environment and working to prevent child sexual abuse.
- Assist employees/volunteers in learning to interact with youth with care and concern in order to foster youth development.

Handling disclosures

Employees/volunteers need to be able to respond appropriately to the person making the disclosure.

- Teach employees/volunteers what they should and should not say to a victim who is disclosing child sexual abuse.
- Instruct employees/volunteers to report sexual abuse allegations, suspicious, and disclosures to the authorities according to your organization's policies. (See "Reporting Process" on page 18.)
- Seek the counsel of the nearest child advocacy center for advice on training about these matters.

Immunity and support for reporters

Employees/volunteers need to know whether they are immune from civil or criminal liability when making a required or authorized report of known or suspected child sexual abuse.

- Check with state laws on whether employees/volunteers are immune from civil or criminal liability when making a report.
- Share immunity information with employees/volunteers.
- Reassure employees/volunteers that they will be supported by your organization and its management in their efforts to protect youth and that debriefing and/or counseling will be available to reporters and bystanders should abuse occur.

Training Caregivers

Two main areas of education should be emphasized with caregivers (i.e., parents and guardians) of youth in youth-serving organizations: (1) education specific to child sexual abuse and (2) education about the organization's child sexual abuse prevention policies and procedures.

Critical Content for Training Caregivers

Child sexual abuse information

Caregivers need to understand child sexual abuse and their role in preventing it. Education in this area should be in the context of explaining healthy sexual development (e.g., what is appropriate and when).

- Define child sexual abuse, including the continuum of appropriate, inappropriate, and harmful behaviors.
- Challenge commonly held myths about child sexual abuse, such as the myth that most offenders are strangers and are easily identifiable.
- Describe warning signs for sexually offending behaviors and victimization (i.e., what to watch for).
- Discuss how to talk to their children about sexuality and child sexual abuse as well as how to talk to other adults about child sexual abuse both before and after any suspicion of sexual abuse has been raised. Use role playing to make caregivers feel more comfortable bringing up these topics.
- Explain caregivers' responsibility to act if they witness or hear about inappropriate or harmful behaviors.
- Describe where to go for help within your organization, such as who the point person for child sexual abuse is inside your organization.
- Provide resources for seeking help outside your organization, such as child sexual abuse prevention organizations. (See "Resource List and Sample Policies" in Appendix B.)

Organization's child sexual abuse policies and procedures

Caregivers should be informed about your organization's child sexual abuse prevention policies and procedures so they know what your organization expects of them and what they can expect of your organization and its employees/volunteers.

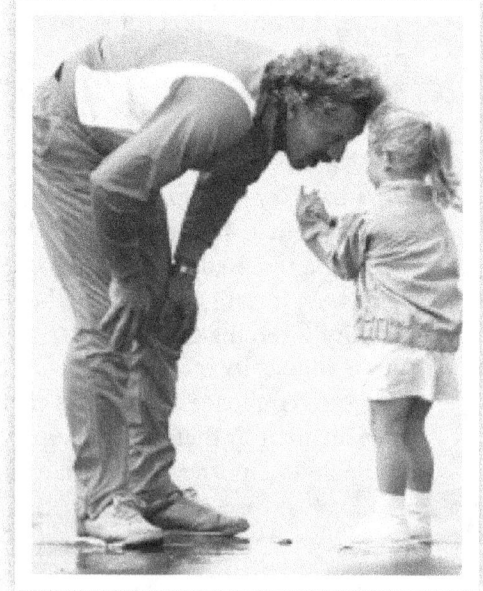

- Describe what your organization does, such as its mission and role.
- Define what activities are appropriate and inappropriate in your organization, such as whether your organization sponsors overnight trips, mentoring, or one-on-one coaching.
- Delineate responsibilities of the caregiver and your organization. For example, define who is responsible for transporting youth.
- Encourage caregivers to attend sessions and programs whenever they can to make sure that youth are being protected and that policies are being followed.

Training Youth

Child sexual abuse education and training for youth should be both developmentally appropriate and at the proper skill level. For example, different skills and knowledge may be provided to adolescents and younger children.

Critical Content for Training Youth

Child sexual abuse information

Your organization needs to provide youth with some basic child sexual abuse information.

- Provide general information about child sexual abuse, including what constitutes appropriate, inappropriate, and harmful behavior from adults and other youth. For example, youth need to know that no one has the right to force, trick, or coerce them into sexual situations and that sexual offenders, not their victims, are responsible for their behavior.
- Teach youth how to interact appropriately with each other.
- Discuss the importance of reporting sexual abuse.
- Tell youth to whom they should report what they believe is inappropriate or harmful behavior.
- Seek assistance from other organizations that have created personal safety programs if your organization is interested in implementing one.

Protective factors

There are factors that can help prevent youth from getting sexually abused or abusing. Youth should be educated about how they can make themselves and others safer.

- Educate youth about the bystander approach. Empower youth to intervene or tell someone when they see inappropriate or harmful interactions between adults and youth or between youth. Encourage youth to tell a trusted adult about inappropriate or harmful things that have happened to themselves or their friends.

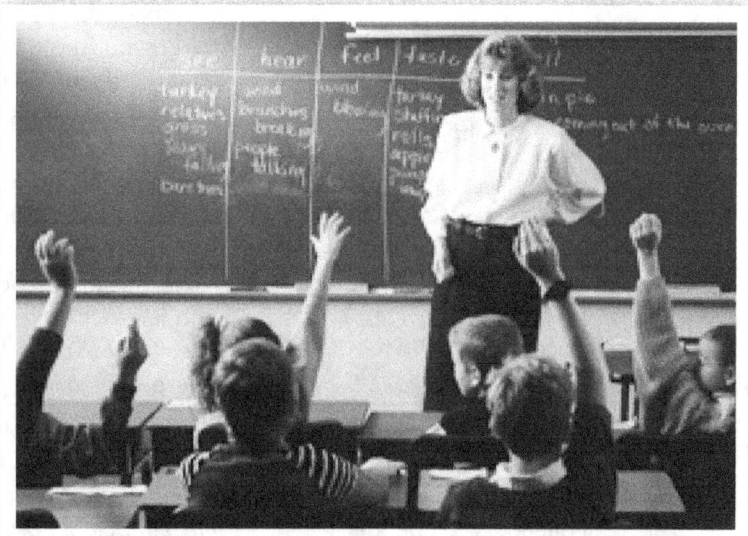

- Empower youth as partners in the prevention process. Encourage them to adopt healthy strategies to protect themselves, such as checking with a caregiver/adult before doing activities, going places with friends instead of alone, and identifying trusted adults.
- Educate youth about healthy sexuality. Teach youth to recognize appropriate behavior and to avoid exploitive or inappropriate behavior toward others.

Overcoming Challenges to Child Sexual Abuse Prevention in Youth-serving Organizations

Organizations that are committed to preventing child sexual abuse will likely face challenges in implementing prevention policies and strategies. Which challenges an organization faces will depend largely on its type, size, and level of commitment to child sexual abuse prevention. Not all challenges described in this document will apply to your organization. Awareness of potential challenges, however, will better prepare you for such encounters.

Most challenges that organizations face in child sexual abuse prevention fall into two broad categories: beliefs and structural issues.

The following tables present some of the challenges within these categories and suggest some of the strategies that organizations have used to overcome them.

Table 1. Beliefs that hinder child sexual abuse prevention

Challenges	Strategies to Overcome Challenges
Beliefs that hinder child sexual abuse prevention	*Overall strategy for overcoming belief challenge: good training* • Instructors/supervisors: Ensure that well-trained, approachable instructors and supervisors can promote positive communication, answer questions, and demonstrate how strategies will help make youth and employees/volunteers safer. Make sure that consistent messages are conveyed by these individuals. • Environment: Training effectiveness is greatly enhanced when a safe environment is created so that employees/volunteers feel free to ask questions. • Mechanism/interactivity: Accessible (e.g., online) and interactive training methods can be used to effectively change beliefs that hinder child sexual abuse prevention.
Denial related to child sexual abuse • Belief that child sexual abuse never happens in "my organization." • Belief that offenders can be identified by a stereotype (e.g., offenders are "monsters" and not the nice employees/volunteers that you know in your organization).	• Use *statistics* to justify your organization's efforts. • Use *current events* to highlight the need for child sexual abuse prevention within your organization. • *Present actual cases* (i.e., personal stories) to make people aware of the need for child sexual abuse prevention and to show that offenders are not easily identified by stereotypes.

Fear that people will think something is wrong within your organization because it is focusing on the issue of child sexual abuse.	The way that your organization *frames* child sexual abuse prevention can make all the difference in overcoming this challenge. Experts suggest that organizations use the following frames when discussing your efforts to prevent child sexual abuse: • Child sexual abuse prevention efforts enhance your organization's mission to nurture and protect youth. • The well-being of youth (including their freedom from child sexual abuse) is part of your organizational mission. • Policies to protect youth also protect your organization and the employees/volunteers who work there. • Organizations that are proactive about child sexual abuse prevention show corporate responsibility. • Prevention of child sexual abuse is only one area of youth safety about which your organization is concerned.
Attitudes about sexuality • A cultural reluctance to talk about sex and child sexual abuse. • A belief that it is not your organization's place to deal with child sexual abuse.	Because this challenge applies not just to organizations but to our culture as a whole, this challenge is particularly difficult to overcome. *Make sure that these issues get discussed regularly in your organization, especially in training.* Also involve caregivers and other stakeholders in these discussions. Over time, perseverance and open communication should overcome this barrier.
Denial and fear can result in lack of buy-in from all levels of employees/ volunteers. Some organizations are challenged by a lack of support for this issue from management and an unwillingness of employees/volunteers to spend time on child sexual abuse prevention. This is particularly true when child sexual abuse prevention is not identified as a high priority in organizations.	*Be persistent* in addressing myths, denial, and fear related to child sexual abuse prevention. Continue to train all levels of employees/volunteers about the importance of this issue.
Fear of uncovering child sexual abuse cases when adopting child sexual abuse prevention strategies.	When your organization adopts child sexual abuse prevention strategies and policies, you may initially encounter an increase in the number of disclosures of child sexual abuse. This is because the strategies are uncovering cases that have been hidden. *The hope is that once these cases have been uncovered and prevention strategies are consistently implemented, the number of reported cases will decrease.*

Table 2: Structural issues that hinder child sexual abuse prevention

Challenges	Strategies to Overcome Challenges
Structural issues that hinder child sexual abuse prevention	*Overall strategy for overcoming structural issues challenge: leadership* Strong leadership within your organization that emphasizes the importance of child sexual abuse prevention can help make some challenging structural issues more manageable. One essential way that your leadership can emphasize your dedication to child sexual abuse prevention is to designate a point of contact for child sexual abuse prevention, while reiterating that everyone in your organization is responsible for prevention. This point of contact needs to be someone with enough expertise and training to answer questions and spearhead your organization's policies. If your organization is multilayered or large, you can designate people at different levels to do this work. Dedicating staff to this issue, even if part-time, can make dealing with structural issues much easier.
Limited/inadequate resources • Lack of money • Lack of time • Lack of personnel • Lack of expertise	*Many of the strategies recommended cost little or nothing.* For example, training and education content can be added to existing education and accessing community or state experts can help provide expertise. For strategies that require funding, your organization should consider *seeking outside funding for implementation.* For example, consider applying for grants for developing a policy, making environmental changes, or hiring someone to coordinate child sexual abuse prevention efforts.
Poor employee/volunteer retention can make it very difficult to implement child sexual abuse policies because your organization needs to constantly screen, train, and orient new employees/volunteers. These difficulties may be caused by the seasonality of employees/volunteers (e.g., at camps) or simply by a high turnover of employees/volunteers. Other retention issues that may inhibit your organization from adopting child sexual abuse prevention strategies include the fear that much-needed volunteers will not want to go through the screening process and the nature of compassion fatigue (i.e., people just want to be employees/volunteers and do not want to deal with child sexual abuse and/or other difficult topics).	To overcome this challenge, the importance of *ongoing and frequent training* cannot be overemphasized. Regularly scheduled training sessions should be complemented by the incorporation of training and supervision into everyday work. In addition, to combat some fears that you may have about employee/volunteer reluctance to engage in child sexual abuse prevention, *explain to all applicants and employees/volunteers the reasoning behind the screening process and child sexual abuse prevention policies*—they are a piece of your organization's mission to make youth safer. Understanding the motivation behind your efforts may make individuals more willing to participate.

Tendency to rely on one strategy (e.g., criminal background checks) as the sole effort in child sexual abuse prevention.	The first step to combating this tendency is to *read this document*. Then, *have conversations with other organizations*, which will enable you to see that child sexual abuse prevention, like other safety promotion strategies, requires many efforts at multiple levels to make up a comprehensive prevention approach. There is no single, simple way to prevent child sexual abuse.
Difficulty of adoption of the child sexual abuse prevention policy and efforts within your organization can be caused by problems with internal communication (i.e., what gets communicated within your organization) and complicated control mechanisms (i.e., who dictates what is mandatory within your organization).	*Clear and consistent communication* about child sexual abuse issues can help increase adoption within your organization. Create open lines of communication about child sexual abuse prevention within your organization and between your organization and its stakeholders (e.g., caregivers).
Your organization does not know what help is available to develop and implement child sexual abuse prevention strategies.	*Partnerships* are important in overcoming this challenge. Some ideas for partnership include the following: • Work with organization(s) with expertise in implementing child sexual abuse prevention policies and procedures. • Talk with organizations about their child sexual abuse prevention strategies and how they overcame challenges. • Discuss policies with child protective services and law enforcement to make sure they are consistent and appropriate. Ally with these organizations before any allegations or suspicions of child sexual abuse arise. • Use children's advocacy centers, your state sexual violence coalition, your local rape crisis center, and the National Sexual Violence Resource Center as resources. Refer to the "Resource List and Sample Policies" section for more information (Appendix B).

Conclusion: Moving Forward

Implementing a child sexual abuse prevention policy and making the changes necessary to protect youth from child sexual abuse in organizations are not easy tasks. Although organizations should take on as many individual strategies to prevent child sexual abuse as they are able, organizations must have a strong infrastructure in place to serve as a foundation for efforts to prevent child sexual abuse. In addition, because the number of recommended child sexual abuse prevention strategies can be overwhelming, organizations should use the planning tool provided at the end of this

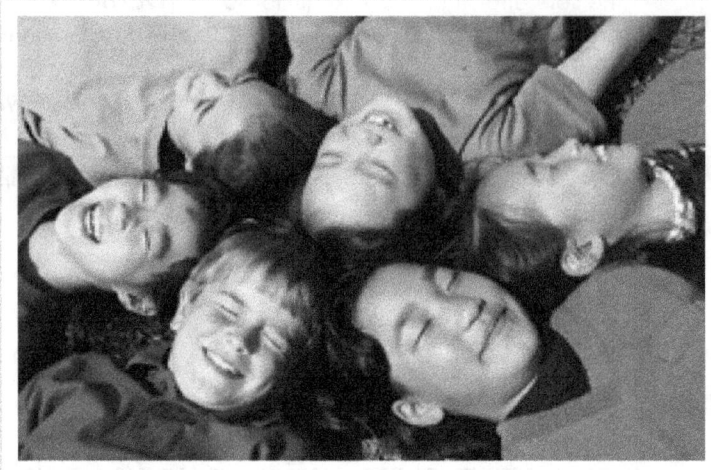

section to help prioritize their efforts. If your organization is committed to preventing child sexual abuse and takes this charge on thoughtfully and with careful planning, it can and will succeed in creating a safer place for the youth under its care.

Organizational Processes for Developing and Implementing Child Sexual Abuse Prevention Policies

Organizations should take several steps to effectively implement child sexual abuse prevention strategies.

Create a safe space
To ensure the effectiveness of child sexual abuse prevention, your organization needs to create an open environment in which employees/volunteers feel comfortable discussing child sexual abuse.

Have clear goals
When deciding what child sexual abuse prevention policies and practices to implement in your organization, always identify clear goals.
- Know why a certain strategy, policy, or practice is being considered and/or adopted to ensure that the most effective means are used to obtain goals.

Create a process for developing child sexual abuse prevention policies and practices
This involves obtaining buy-in from all levels of your organization so that policies and practices are accepted and owned by everyone. All processes can be specific to child sexual abuse planning or may be integrated into a current risk management planning process.
- Develop the policy. For example, gather a group of stakeholders, such as caregivers, employees/volunteers, and attorneys, to do the work.
- Approve the policy, which includes making sure it complies with organizational policies, state and national laws, and child protective services and law enforcement.
- Adopt the policy.

- Develop a system to track allegations of child sexual abuse and outcomes of cases. (See "Internal records" on page 19.)
- Inform your organization about the policy.
- Implement the policy.
- Evaluate the policy to continuously measure whether goals are being met. For example, the goal of setting criteria for screening and selection of employees/volunteers may be to make sure that employees/volunteers are appropriate for working with the youth within your organization. Once that goal is agreed upon and the screening and selection policies are adopted, your organization needs to reassess on a regular basis if that goal is being met. If it is not, what needs to be changed to meet the goal? If it is, consider more efficient ways to meet the goal.

Include appropriate child sexual abuse polices and practices in the prevention plan
In choosing child sexual abuse prevention policies and practices to adopt, your organization should gather information from several sources.
- Consider the strategies raised in this document.
- Use other organizations' experiences in this area. For example, look at the resources and sample policies included in the "Resource List and Sample Policies" section. (See Appendix B.) You may also consider discussing prevention policies with other organizations.

Child Sexual Abuse Prevention Planning Tool for Organizations

This checklist can help your organization plan child sexual abuse prevention efforts in the next year and beyond. It summarizes the critical strategies discussed in this document. Because so many of the additional strategies to consider were specific to certain types of organizations, these are not included in the matrix. Space has been left at the bottom of the tool to add additional strategies.

Child sexual abuse prevention component	Strategy	Page where strategy can be found	Done/in place	Short term (next 12 months)	Long term (3-5 years)	Not applicable to my organization
Screening and selecting of employees/volunteers	Education about organization and youth-protection policies	4				
	Written application	5				
	Personal interview	5				
	Reference checks	7				
	Criminal background checks	7				
Guidelines on interactions between individuals	Appropriate/inappropriate/harmful behaviors	9				
	Ratios of employees/volunteers to youth	9				
	One-on-one interactions	11				
	Risk of interactions between youth	11				
	Prohibitions and restrictions on certain activities	11				
	Out-of-program contact restrictions	11				
	Caregiver information and permission	12				

Child sexual abuse prevention component	Strategy	Page where strategy can be found	Done/ in place	Short term (next 12 months)	Long term (3-5 years)	Not applicable to my organiza-tion
	Responsibility for youth	12				
Monitoring behavior	Responding to what is observed	13				
	Roles and responsibilities	13				
	Clear reporting structure within organization	14				
	Observation and contact with employees/ volunteers	14				
	Documentation that monitoring has occurred	14				
Ensuring safe environments	Visibility	15				
	Privacy when toileting, showering, changing clothes	15				
	Access control	15				
	Off-site activity guidelines	16				
	Transportation policies	16				
Responding to inappropriate behavior, breaches in policy, and allegations and suspicions of child sexual abuse	What to respond to and what to report	17				

Child sexual abuse prevention component	Strategy	Page where strategy can be found	Done/ in place	Short term (next 12 months)	Long term (3-5 years)	Not applicable to my organiza- tion
	Reporting process	18				
	Internal records	19				
	Confidentiality policy	20				
	Response to the press and the community	20				
	Membership/ employment of alleged offenders	20				
Training employees/ volunteers	All policies and procedures organization chooses	24				
	Child sexual abuse information	24				
	Importance of preventing child sexual abuse	25				
	Personal conduct	25				
	Healthy development of youth	25				
	Protective factors	26				
	Handling disclosures	26				
	Immunity and support for reporters	26				
Training caregivers	Child sexual abuse information	27				
	Organization's child sexual abuse policies and procedures	27				

Child sexual abuse prevention component	Strategy	Page where strategy can be found	Done/ in place	Short term (next 12 months)	Long term (3-5 years)	Not applicable to my organiza- tion
Training youth	Child sexual abuse information	28				
	Protective factors	28				
Additional strategies to consider						

Appendix A
Participant List

American Camp Association
(www.acacamps.org)
Patricia Hammond
Formerly Director of Standards

Current representative: Wes Bird
Director of Accreditation Programs
American Camp Association
5000 State Rd. 67 North
Martinsville, IN 46151-7902
Phone: 765-342-8456, ext. 306
E-mail: wbird@acacamps.org

American Youth Soccer Organization
(www.soccer.org)
Ellisa Hall
12501 S. Isis Ave.
Hawthorne, CA 90250
Phone: 800-872-2976 x 361
E-mail: EllisaHall@ayso.org

Big Brothers Big Sisters of America
(www.bbbs.org)
Julie Novak
Director of Child Safety and Quality Assurance
E4337 Spruce Rd.
Eleva, WI 54738
Phone: 715-878-9670
E-mail: jnovak@bbbs.org

Joseph Radelet, Ed.D.
Vice President, Mentoring Program
230 North 13th St.
Philadelphia, PA 19107-1538
Phone: 215-665-7768
Fax: 215-567-0394
E-mail: jradelet@bbbs.org

Boys & Girls Clubs of America
(www.kidbuilding.org)
R. Leslie Nichols, AIA
Vice President, Club Safety & Design
1230 W. Peachtree St., NW
Atlanta, GA 30309
Phone: 404-487-5746
Fax: 404-487-5969
E-mail: lnichols@bcga.org

Boy Scouts of America
(www.scouting.org)
Current representative: James J. Terry
National Director of Administration
Administration Group National Office
1325 West Walnut Hill Ln.
P.O. Box 152079
Irving, TX 75015-2079
Phone: 972-580-2225
Fax: 972-580-7849
E-mail: jterry@netbsa.org

Crimes against Children Research Center,
University of New Hampshire
(www.unh.edu/ccrc/)
David Finkelhor, Ph.D.
Family Research Laboratory
Department of Sociology
University of New Hampshire
Durham, NH 03824
Phone: 603-862-2761
Fax: 603-862-1122
E-mail: david.finkelhor@unh.edu

Darkness to Light
(www.d2l.org)
Trisha Folds Bennett, Ph.D.
Director of Programs Products and Services
7 Radcliffe St., Suite 200
Charleston, SC 29403
Phone: 843-965-5444
Fax: 843-965-5449
E-mail: tbennett@d2l.org

National School Boards Association
(www.nsba.org)
Brenda Z. Greene
Director of School Health Programs
1680 Duke St.
Alexandria, VA 22314
Phone: 703 838-6756
Fax: 703-548-5516
E-mail: bgreene@nsba.org

National Sexual Violence Resource Center
(www.nsvrc.org)
Karen Baker, L.M.S.W.
123 N. Enola Dr.
Enola, PA 17025
Toll-free phone: 877-739-3895
Fax: 717-909-0714
E-mail: kbaker@nsvrc.org

Nonprofit Risk Management Center
(www.nonprofitrisk.org)
John Patterson
Senior Program Director
1130 Seventeenth St., NW, Suite 210
Washington, DC 20036
Phone: 202-785-3891
Fax: 202-296-0349
E-mail: John@nonprofitrisk.org

Portland State University
Keith Kaufman, Ph.D.
Professor and Department Chair
Psychology Department
P.O. Box 751
Portland, OR 97207-0751
Phone: 503-725-3984
Fax: 503-725-3904
E-mail: kaufmank@pdx.edu

Sensibilities, Inc.
Cordelia Anderson
4405 Garfield Ave. South
Minneapolis, MN 55409
Phone: 612-824-6217
Fax: 612-824-6930
E-mail: Cordelia@visi.com

Special Olympics, Inc.
(www.specialolympics.org)
Dave Lenox
1133 19th St., NW
Washington, DC 20036
Phone: 202-628-3630
E-mail: dlenox@specialolympics.org

Stop it NOW!
(www.stopitnow.org)
Joan Tabachnick
Formerly Director of Public Education

Current representative: Peter Pollard
351 Pleasant St., Suite B319
Northampton, MA 01060
Phone: 413-587-3500, ext. 14
Fax: 413-587-3505
E-mail: ppollard@stopitnow.org

Union for Reform Judaism Camps
(www.urjcamps.org)
Rabbi Glynis Conyer
Formerly Director of Staff Development &
Training

Current representative: David Berkman
Associate Director of Camping
Union for Reform Judaism
633 Third Ave., 7th Floor
New York, NY 10017
Phone: 212-650-4216
Fax: 212-650-4199
E-mail: dberkman@urj.org

Unitarian Universalist Association
of Congregations
(www.uua.org)
Rev. Patricia Hoertdoerfer
Formerly Children's Program and Family
Ministry Director

Current representative: Tracey Robinson-Harris
UUA Office of Ethics and Safety
25 Beacon St.
Boston, MA 02018
Phone: 617-948-6462
Fax: 617-742-0321
E-mail: trobinsonharris@uua.org

United Methodist Church
(www.flumc.org)
Carol Sue Hutchinson
Florida Conference
P.O. Box 3767
Lakeland, FL 33802-3767
Phone: 863-688-5563 x 140
Fax: 863-686-7363
E-mail: chutchinson@flumc.org

CDC Participants:
Centers for Disease Control and Prevention
National Center for Injury Prevention
  and Control
Division of Violence Prevention
4770 Buford Hwy., NE, Mailstop K-60
Atlanta, GA 30341
Website: www.cdc.gov/injury

Natalie Audage, M.P.H.
Consultant and former ASPH/CDC Fellow

Corinne Graffunder, M.P.H.
Branch Chief
Program Implementation and
  Dissemination Branch

Janet Saul, Ph.D.
Branch Chief
Prevention Development and
  Evaluation Branch

Appendix B
Resource List and Sample Policies

Books/Publications/Videos/Worksops Related to Child Sexual Abuse Prevention

X indicates discussion topics.

Book/Publication/Video/Workshop	Screening and selecting employees/ volunteers	Guidelines on interactions between individuals	Monitoring behavior	Ensuring safe environments	Responding	Training employees/ volunteers	Training caregivers/ youth	General/ overall
Accreditation Standards for Camp Programs and Services American Camp Association; 1998. Has sample staff application form and voluntary disclosure form. (www.acacamps.org)	X	X	X					X
The APSAC Handbook of Child Maltreatment (2nd Edition) John E.B. Myers, Lucy Berliner, John Briere, C. Terry Hendrix, Carole Jenny, Theresa A. Reid, editors Sage Publications; 2002.								X
Balancing Acts: Keeping Children Safe in Congregations Reverend Debra Haffner Unitarian Universalist Association; 2005. (www.uua.org/cde/ethics/balancing/)							X	X
Basic Camp Management: An Introduction to Camp Administration Armand and Beverly Ball American Camp Association; 2004. (www.acacamps.org)	X	X	X	X	X	X		
Being Smart, Playing Safe: New Guidelines for Counselor Behavior (video) Bob Ditter American Camp Association; 2003. (www.acacamps.org)		X				X		X

Book/Publication/Video/Workshop	Screening and selecting employees/ volunteers	Guidelines on interactions between individuals	Monitoring behavior	Ensuring safe environments	Responding	Training employees/ volunteers	Training caregivers/ youth	General/ overall
Creating Safe Congregations: Toward an Ethic of Right Relations Workbook Patricia Hoertdoerfer and William Sinkford, editors Unitarian Universalist Association; 1997.		X		X				X
Flirting or Hurting: Teachers' Guide to Student-to-Student Sexual Harassment in Schools Nan Stein and Lisa Sjostrom National Education Association; 1994.		X		X				X
For Their Sake: Recognizing, Responding to, and Reporting Child Abuse Becca Cowan Johnson American Camp Association; 1992. A staff training handbook is also available. (www.acacamps.org)			X		X	X	X	X
Hysteria Management: Child Abuse and Camp (video) Bob Ditter American Camp Association; 1989. (www.acacamps.org)						X	X	X
Identifying Child Molesters: Preventing Child Sexual Abuse by Recognizing the Patterns of the Offenders Carla van Dam Haworth Maltreatment and Trauma Press; 2001.		X				X	X	X
The Juvenile Sexual Offender Howard E. Barbaree, William L. Marshall, Stephen M. Hudson Guilford; 1993.								X

Book/Publication/Video/Workshop	Screening and selecting employees/volunteers	Guidelines on interactions between individuals	Monitoring behavior	Ensuring safe environments	Responding	Training employees/volunteers	Training caregivers/youth	General/overall
The Little Book on Restorative Justice Howard Zehr Good Books; 2002.								X
Nursery Crimes: Sexual Abuse in Day Care David Finkelhor, Linda Meyer Williams, Nanci Burns, Michael Kalinowski Sage Publications; 1988.								X
Our Whole Lives curricula Unitarian Universalist Association (www.uua.org/owl/) *Our Whole Lives Grades K–1* Barbara Sprung; 2000. *Our Whole Lives Grades 4–6* Elizabeth Casparian and Eva Goldfarb; 2000. *Our Whole Lives Grades 7–9* Pamela Wilson; 1999. *Our Whole Lives Grades 10–12* Eva Goldfarb and Elizabeth Casparian; 2000. *Our Whole Lives Adult* Richard Kimball; 2000.		X				X	X	X
Peacemaking Circles: From Crime to Community Kay Prawis, Barry Stuart, Mark Wedge Living Justice Press; 2003.		X	X					X
Protecting God's Children Program for Adults National Catholic Services, LLC; 2002. (www.virtus.org)	X	X	X		X	X	X (for adults)	X

44

Book/Publication/Video/Workshop	Screening and selecting employees/ volunteers	Guidelines on interactions between individuals	Monitoring behavior	Ensuring safe environments	Responding	Training employees/ volunteers	Training caregivers/ youth	General/ overall
Reducing the Risk II: Making Your Church Safe from Child Sexual Abuse James Cobble, Richard Hammar, Steven Klipowicz Christian Ministry Resources; 2003. Also available: DVD, training manual, online training, and resource center (www.reducingtherisk.com)	X	X	X	X	X	X		X
Responsible Staffing: Helping You Create Safe Congregations for Children, Youth, and Vulnerable Adults Unitarian Universalist Association; 2000. (www.uua.org/programs/ministry/responsiblestaffing.html)	X	X	X	X	X	X		X
Safe Congregations Handbook: Nurturing Healthy Boundaries in Our Faith Communities Patricia Hoertdoerfer and Fredric Muir Unitarian Universalist Association; 2005. (www.uua.org)	X	X	X	X	X	X	X	X
Safe Sanctuaries for Youth: Reducing the Risk of Abuse in Youth Ministries Joy Thornburg Melton Discipleship Resources; 2003. Also available: DVD (www.upperroom.org)	X	X	X	X	X	X	X	X
Screening Volunteers to Prevent Child Sexual Abuse: A Community Guide for Youth Organizations American Camp Association; 1997. (www.acacamps.org)	X							

Book/Publication/Video/Workshop	Screening and selecting employees/volunteers	Guidelines on interactions between individuals	Monitoring behavior	Ensuring safe environments	Responding	Training employees/volunteers	Training caregivers/youth	General/overall
The Season of Hope: A Risk Management Guide for Youth-Serving Nonprofits John Patterson and Barbara Oliver Nonprofit Risk Management Center; 2002. (www.nonprofitrisk.org)	X	X	X	X	X	X		X
Smarter Adults-Safer Children program AGOS (developed for National Catholic Services, LLC); 2004. (www.agosnet.com)	X	X	X		X	X	X (for adults)	X
Spoilsports: Understanding and Preventing Sexual Exploitation in Sport Celia H. Brackenridge Routledge; 2001.	X							X
Staff Screening Tool Kit, 3rd Edition Nonprofit Risk Management Center; 2004. (www.nonprofitrisk.org)	X							
Stewards of Children: Adults Resolving Child Sexual Abuse in Community Darkness to Light Curriculum; 2004. (www.d2l.org)	X	X			X	X	X (for caregivers only)	X
A Time to Heal: Protecting Children and Ministering to Sex Offenders Reverend Debra Haffner Christian Community and LifeQuest; 2005.							X	X
What Do I Do Now? Challenges and Choices for Camp Counselors and Other Youth Leaders Jerome Beker, Doug Magnunson, Connie Magnunson, David Beker American Camp Association; 1996. Includes case studies and scenarios. (www.acacamps.org)								X

Journal Articles

Finkelhor D. Four preconditions: a model. In: Finkelhor D, editor. *Child sexual abuse: new theory and research*. New York (NY): The Free Press; 1984. p. 53–68.

Kaufman K, Hilliker D, Daleiden E. Subgroup differences in the modus operandi of adolescent sexual offenders. *Child Maltreatment* 1996;1(1):17–24.

Kaufman K, Holmberg J, Orts K, McCrady F, Rotzien A, Daleiden E, et al. Factors influencing sexual offenders' modus operandi: an examination of victim-offender relatedness and age. *Child Maltreatment* 1998;3(4):349–61.

Kenny MC, McEachem AG. Racial, ethnic, and cultural factors of childhood sexual abuse: a selected review of the literature. *Clinical Psychology Review* 2000;20(7):905–22.

Mesuraco B. Primary preventive intervention in a modern and diverse society. *Australian and New Zealand Journal of Family Therapy* 2002; 23(1):33–7.

Millan F, Robiner SS. Toward a culturally sensitive child sexual abuse prevention program for Latinos. *Journal of Social Distress and the Homeless* 1992;1(3/4): 311–20.

Ryan G. Childhood sexuality: a decade of study. Part 1-research and current development. *Child Abuse and Neglect* 2000;1:33–48.

Sample Policies from Participating Organizations

American Youth Soccer Organization
- Go to www.soccer.org.
- Click on AYSO PROGRAMS on the top tab.
- Click on Safe Haven in the left pull-down menu.
- Click on Safe Haven Resources in the expanded Safe Haven menu.

Boy Scouts of America
- Go to www.scouting.org/pubs/ypt/resources.html.

Florida Conference of the United Methodist Church
- Go to www.flumc.org.
- Look under the Administration tab for "Child Protection Policy."

National Catholic Services, LLC
- Go to www.virtus.org.
- Click on "Pastoral Conduct," "Volunteer Conduct," and "Response to Allegations" under "Model Policies" on the left menu.

Unitarian Universalist Association
- Go to www.uua.org/cde/education/safecong.html.
- The home page for Ethics and Safety is www.uua.org/cde/ethics.

Publications with Sample Policies and Procedures

Accreditation Standards for Camp Programs and Services
American Camp Association; 1998.
Includes sample staff application form and voluntary disclosure form
www.acacamps.org

Responsible Staffing: Helping You Create Safe Congregations for Children, Youth, and Vulnerable Adults
Unitarian Universalist Association; 2000.
Includes guidelines for screening, sample forms for reference checks, and sample volunteer application form
www.uua.org/programs/ministry/responsiblestaffing.html

Safe Sanctuaries for Youth: Reducing the Risk of Abuse in Youth Ministries
Joy Thornburg Melton
Discipleship resources; 2003.
Includes sample screening forms and sample youth abuse prevention policy

The Season of Hope: A Risk Management Guide for Youth-Serving Nonprofits
John Patterson and Barbara Oliver
Nonprofit Risk Management Center; 2002.
Includes sample consent form for criminal background checks
www.nonprofitrisk.org

Staff Screening Tool Kit, 3rd Edition
Nonprofit Risk Management Center; 2004.
Includes guidance on screening
www.nonprofitrisk.org

Relevant Organizations

American Camp Association
www.acacamps.org

American Youth Soccer Organization
www.soccer.org

Big Brothers Big Sisters of America
www.bbbs.org

Boys & Girls Clubs of America
www.kidbuilding.org

Boy Scouts of America
www.scouting.org

Centers for Disease Control and Prevention
www.cdc.gov/injury

Child Advocacy Centers
www.nca-online.org

Crimes against Children Research Center, University of New Hampshire
www.unh.edu/ccrc/

Darkness to Light
www.d2l.org

FaithTrust Institute
www.faithtrustinstitute.org

FBI State Sex Offender Registries
www.fbi.gov/hq/cid/cac/states.htm

Minnesota Center Against Violence and Abuse
www.mincava.umn.edu

National Center for Missing and Exploited Children
www.missingkids.com
www.cybertipline.com

National School Boards Association
www.nsba.org

National Sexual Violence Resource Center
www.nsvrc.org

Nonprofit Risk Management Center
www.nonprofitrisk.org

Prevent Child Abuse America
www.preventchildabuse.org

Sexuality Information and Education Council of the U.S.
www.siecus.org

Special Olympics, Inc.
www.specialolympics.org

Stop it NOW!
www.stopitnow.org

Union for Reform Judaism Camps
www.urjcamps.org

Unitarian Universalist Association of Congregations
www.uua.org

United Methodist Church-Florida Conference
www.flumc.org

Your State's Sexual Violence Coalition
www.nsvrc.org/resources/orgs/coalitions/index.html

CS107800

For more information:

Centers for Disease Control and Prevention
National Center for Injury Prevention and Control
1-800-CDC-INFO • www.cdc.gov/injury • CDCinfo@cdc.gov

CS107800

www.ingramcontent.com/pod-product-compliance
Lightning Source LLC
Chambersburg PA
CBHW081904170526
45167CB00007B/3138